1

Contents

4

chronic kidney disease

Chronic kidney disease (CKD) is a long-term condition where the kidneys do not work effectively.

CKD does not usually cause symptoms until it reaches an advanced stage. It is usually detected at earlier stages by blood and urine tests. Main symptoms of advanced kidney disease include:

- tiredness
- swollen ankles, feet or hands (due to water retention)
- shortness of breath
- nausea
- blood in the urine

Chronic kidney disease is most frequently diagnosed through blood and urine tests.

If you are at a high risk of developing CKD, you may be screened annually. Screening may be recommended if you have:

- high blood pressure (hypertension)
- diabetes
- a family history of CKD

Why does it happen?

The kidneys are two bean-shaped organs, the size of your fist, located on either side of the body, just beneath the ribcage. The main role of the kidneys is to filter waste products from the blood before converting them into urine. The kidneys also:

- help maintain blood pressure
- maintain the correct levels of chemicals in your body which, in turn, will help heart and muscles function properly
- produce the active form of vitamin D that keeps bones healthy
- produce a substance called erythropoietin, which stimulates production of red blood cells

Chronic kidney disease is the reduced ability of the kidney to carry out these functions in the long-term. This is most often caused by damage to the kidneys from other conditions, most commonly diabetes and high blood pressure.

Who is affected?

CKD is common and mainly associated with ageing. The older you get, the more likely you are to have some degree of kidney disease.

It is estimated that about one in five men and one in four women between the ages of 65 and 74 has some degree of CKD.

CKD is more common in people of south Asian origin (those from India, Bangladesh, Sri Lanka and Pakistan) and black people than the general population. The reasons for this include higher rates of diabetes in south Asian people and higher rates of high blood pressure in African or Caribbean people.

Treating chronic kidney disease

There is no cure for chronic kidney disease, although treatment can slow or halt the progression of the disease and can prevent other serious conditions developing.

People with CKD are known to have an increased risk of a heart attack because of changes that occur to the circulation.

In a minority of people, CKD may cause kidney failure, also known as established renal failure (ERF) or end-stage kidney disease. In this situation, the usual functions of the kidney stop working.

To survive, people with ERF may need to have artificial kidney treatment, called dialysis, or a kidney transplant.

Being diagnosed with chronic kidney disease can be worrying, but support and advice are available to help you cope.

Preventing chronic kidney disease

The main way to reduce the chances of CKD developing is to ensure any existing conditions, such as diabetes and high blood pressure, are carefully managed.

Some lifestyle changes can also reduce the risk of CKD developing, these include:

- having a healthy diet
- avoiding drinking excessive amounts of alcohol
- exercising regularly
- avoiding medicines that can damage the kidney

Symptoms of chronic kidney disease

Most people with CKD have no symptoms because the body can tolerate even a large reduction in kidney function.

In other words, we are born with a lot more kidney function than is necessary for survival. Kidney function is often sufficient if only one kidney is working. That is why people can give a kidney to someone needing a kidney transplant.

A change in kidney function is usually discovered through a routine blood or urine test. If you are diagnosed with kidney disease, your kidney function will be monitored with regular blood and urine tests, and treatment aims to keep any symptoms to a minimum.

If the kidneys continue to lose function and there is progression towards kidney failure (established renal failure or ERF), this will usually be tracked by blood tests and monitoring. If kidney failure does occur, the symptoms may include:

- weight loss and poor appetite

- swollen ankles, feet or hands (due to water retention)

- shortness of breath

- blood or protein in your urine (protein in your urine is not something you will notice as it can only be detected during a urine test)

- an increased need to urinate, particularly at night

- insomnia

- itchy skin

- muscle cramps

- high blood pressure (hypertension)

- nausea

- erectile dysfunction in men (an inability to get or maintain an erection)

These are general symptoms and can be caused by many less serious conditions. Many of the symptoms above can be avoided if treatment begins at an early stage, before any symptoms appear.

Causes of chronic kidney disease

Kidney disease is most often caused by other conditions that put a strain on the kidneys.

High blood pressure (hypertension) and diabetes are the most common causes of kidney disease. The evidence indicates that high blood pressure causes just over a quarter of all cases of kidney failure. Diabetes has been established as the cause of around a quarter of all cases.

High blood pressure

Blood pressure is a measure of the pressure your heart generates in your arteries with each pulse. Too much pressure can damage your body's organs, leading to heart disease, stroke and worsening of kidney function.

The cause of around 90% of cases of high blood pressure is unknown, although there appears to be a link between the condition and a person's general health, diet, and lifestyle.

Known risk factors for high blood pressure include:

- age (the risk of developing high blood pressure increases as you get older)
- family history of high blood pressure (the condition seems to run in families)
- being of African-Caribbean or south Asian origin
- obesity
- lack of exercise
- smoking
- excessive alcohol consumption
- high amount of salt in your diet
- high-fat diet
- stress

Hypertension causes damage by putting strain on the small blood vessels in the kidneys. This prevents the filtering process from working properly.

Diabetes

Diabetes is a condition in which the body produces no – or too little – insulin (type 1 diabetes) or has become unable to make effective use of insulin (type 2 diabetes).

Insulin is needed to regulate levels of glucose (sugar) in your blood, preventing the levels going too high after a meal and too low between meals.

If diabetes is poorly controlled, too much glucose can build up in your blood. The glucose can damage the tiny filters in the kidneys, which affects the ability of your kidneys to filter out waste products and fluids.

It is estimated that 20-40% of people with type 1 diabetes will develop kidney disease before they reach 50 years of age. Around 30% of people with type 2 diabetes also show signs of developing kidney damage.

The first sign of diabetic kidney disease is the appearance of low levels of protein in the urine. Therefore, your GP will ask for an annual urine test so any kidney disease can be detected as early as possible.

All people with diabetes should have a kidney check every year. Early detection of kidney dysfunction in diabetes is important because it identifies people at risk or complications, such as eye problems and impotence.

Other causes

There are many other conditions that less commonly cause CKD, including:

- glomerulonephritis (inflammation of the kidney)

- pyelonephritis (infection in the kidney)

- polycystic kidney disease (an inherited condition where both kidneys are larger than normal due to the gradual growth of masses of cysts)

- failure of normal kidney development in an unborn baby while developing in the womb

- systemic lupus erythematosus (a condition of the immune system where the body attacks the kidney as if it were foreign tissue)

- long-term, regular use of medicines, such as lithium and non-steroidal anti-inflammatory drugs (NSAIDs), including aspirin and ibuprofen

- blockages, for example due to kidney stones or prostate disease

Diagnosis of chronic kidney disease

Chronic kidney disease (CKD) is most frequently diagnosed through blood and urine tests.

Screening

If you are in a high-risk group for developing CKD, it is important to be regularly screened for the condition. People who are not in a high-risk group are not normally screened for CKD.

Annual screening is recommended for the following groups:

- people with high blood pressure (hypertension)
- people with diabetes
- people with acute kidney injury caused by medications such as lithium or NSAIDs such as ibuprofen, kidney stones or an enlarged prostate

- people with cardiovascular disease (conditions that affect the heart, arteries and veins, such as coronary heart disease or heart failure)
- people with a family history of stage five CKD (see below for more information about staging) or an inherited kidney disease
- people with diseases that affect several parts of the body and may affect the kidneys, such as systemic lupus erythematosus
- people with blood in the urine (haematuria) or protein in the urine (proteinuria) where there is no known cause
- Your GP can advise you about whether or not you should be screened for CKD.

Most often, the diagnosis of kidney disease is made because a routine blood or urine test indicates the kidneys may not be functioning normally. If this happens, the test is usually repeated to confirm the diagnosis.

Glomerular filtration rate (GFR)

An effective way of assessing how well your kidneys are working is to calculate your glomerular filtration rate (GFR). GFR is a measurement of how many millilitres (ml) of waste fluid your kidneys can filter from the blood in a minute (measured in ml/min). A healthy pair of kidneys should be able to filter more than 90ml/min.

It is difficult to measure the GFR directly, so it is estimated using a formula. The result is called the

27

estimated GFR or eGFR. Calculating your eGFR involves taking a blood sample and measuring the levels of a waste product called creatinine and taking into account your age, gender and ethnic group. The result is similar to the percentage of normal kidney function. For example, an eGFR of 50ml/min equates to 50% kidney function.

The following tests are used to detect proteinuria (protein in the urine)

urine tests – used to see whether there is blood or protein in your urine

albumin and creatinine testing – this is another urine test which compares the amounts of albumin (a protein) and creatinine in your urine. The ratio of the two (the albumin:creatinine ratio or ACR) can be used with eGFR to give doctors a more accurate idea of how the kidneys are functioning

Staging

A six-stage system, based on eGFR levels, is used to describe the progression of CKD. The higher the stage, the more severe the CKD. The six stages are described below.

Stage one (sometimes called G1): the eGFR is normal (above 90 or more), but other testing shows evidence of kidney damage.

Stage two (G2): the eGFR has decreased slightly (60–89), but is still considered to be in the normal range for a young adult.

If you have stage one or two CKD, it is recommended you have annual eGFR tests so the progression of the condition can be carefully monitored.

Stage three is divided into two – stage 3a (G3a) and 3b (G3b). In stage 3a, the eGFR has decreased mildly (45–59) and this is termed a mild to moderate decrease in kidney function and should be checked annually. In stage 3b (G3b) it has decreased moderately (30–44) and is termed a moderate to severe reduction in kidney function and should be checked every six months.

Stage four (G4): the eGFR has reduced severely (15-29). By this time, it is possible you will be experiencing symptoms of CKD. Further testing should be carried out every six months.

Stage five (G5): the kidneys have lost almost all of their function (an eGFR of below 15), which is known as established renal failure. Further testing should be carried out every three months.

However, over time, GFR can fluctuate, so one abnormal test result does not automatically mean you have CKD. A diagnosis of CKD is usually only confirmed if repeated eGFR tests show your eGFR is consistently lower than normal over three months.

Other tests

A number of other tests are also used to assess the levels of damage to your kidneys. These are outlined below:

kidney scans, such as an ultrasound scan, a magnetic resonance imaging (MRI) scan or a computerised tomography (CT) scan – used to find out whether there are any unusual blockages in your urine flow. In cases of advanced kidney disease, the kidneys are shrunken and have an uneven shape

kidney biopsy – a small sample of kidney tissue is taken so that the cells can be examined under a microscope for damage

Treating chronic kidney disease

Lifestyle changes

The following lifestyle changes are known to help reduce your blood pressure and help control CKD:

- stopping smoking

- eating a healthy, low-fat, balanced diet

- restricting your salt intake to less than 6g (0.2oz) a day

- not using over-the-counter nonsteroidal anti-inflammatory drugs (NSAIDs), such as ibuprofen, except when advised to by a medical professional

- moderating your alcohol intake so it is within recommended limits (no more than 3-4 units a day for men and 2-3 units a day for women)
- losing weight if you are overweight or obese
- doing regular exercise for at least 30 minutes a day, five times a week

Medications for high blood pressure

One of the main ways to reduce the progression of kidney damage is to manage high blood pressure. Good control of blood pressure is vital to protect the kidneys.

People with CKD should aim to get their blood pressure down to below 140/90mmHg but if you also have diabetes you should aim to get it down to below 130/80mmHg.

34

There are many types of blood pressure drugs. Medicines called angiotensin converting enzyme (ACE) inhibitors are used to control high blood pressure in people with CKD.

As well as reducing blood pressure around the body and reducing the strain on blood vessels, ACE inhibitors give additional protection to the kidney.

ACE inhibitors include:

ramipril

enalapril

lisinopril

perindopril

Side effects of ACE inhibitors include:

a persistent, dry cough

dizziness

tiredness or weakness

headaches

Most of these side effects should pass within a few days, although some people continue to have a dry cough.

If the side effects of ACE inhibitors are particularly troublesome, you can be given an alternative medication called an angiotensin-II receptor blocker (ARB). This group of medicines includes:

candesartan

eprosartan

irbesartan

azilsartan

olmesartan

temisartan

valsartan

losartan

The side effects of ARBs are uncommon, but can include dizziness.

Both ACE inhibitors and ARBs can cause a reduction in kidney function in some people and increased levels of potassium in the blood, so blood tests will need to be performed after you start treatment and whenever the dose changes. If you are on an ACE inhibitor or ARB and you develop a fever/infection or need medicines for other conditions, it's important to ask your doctor if the ACE inhibitor or ARB needs to be temporarily stopped.

Medication to reduce cholesterol

Studies have shown that people with CKD have a higher risk of cardiovascular disease, including heart attacks and strokes. This is because some of the risk factors for CKD are the same as those for heart attacks and strokes, including high blood pressure and high levels of cholesterol in the blood (atherosclerosis).

Statins are a type of medication used to lower cholesterol levels. Cholesterol causes narrowing of the arteries that can lead to a blockage of the blood supply to the heart (causing a heart attack) or the brain (causing a stroke). Statins work by blocking the effects of an enzyme in your liver (called HMG-CoA reductase), which is used to make cholesterol.

Statins sometimes have mild side effects, including:

constipation

diarrhoea

headaches

abdominal pain

Occasionally, statins can cause muscle pain, weakness and tenderness. If you experience any of these symptoms, contact your GP. You may need to have a blood test or change your treatment.

If you have kidney disease, you may be asked to reduce your daily fluid and salt intake. You may develop a build-up of fluid as your kidneys will not be able to get rid of fluid as well as they did before.

If you are asked to reduce the amount of fluid you drink, you must also take into account fluid in foods, such as soup and yoghurt. Your GP or dietitian can advise you about this.

The excess fluid that occurs as a result of kidney disease often builds up in your ankles or around your lungs. You may also be given diuretics (water tablets), such as furosemide, which will help get rid of the excess fluid from your body.

If you do not have any fluid retention and you have not been told to reduce your fluid intake, there is no need to do so. In fact, it could be harmful in some circumstances.

Anaemia

Many people with stage three, four and five CKD develop anaemia. Anaemia is a condition in which you do not have enough red blood cells. Symptoms of anaemia include:

tiredness

lethargy

shortness of breath (dyspnoea)

palpitations (awareness of heartbeat)

Anaemia can occur because of many other conditions and your doctor will investigate to rule out other possible causes.

Most people with kidney disease will be given iron supplements because iron is needed for the production of red blood cells. To boost iron levels, iron may be given as tablets, such as daily ferrous sulphate tablets, or as occasional intravenous infusions.

If this is not enough to treat anaemia, you may be started on injections of erythropoietin, a hormone which helps your body produce more red blood cells. These injections are often administered into a vein (intravenously) or under the skin (subcutaneously). Examples of these injections include epoetin alfa, beta and zeta, darbepoetin and methoxy polyethylene glycol-epoetin beta.

Want to know more?

NICE: Treating anaemia in people with chronic kidney disease

Correction of phosphate balance

If you have stage four or five kidney disease, you can get a build-up of phosphate in your body because your kidneys cannot get rid of it. Phosphate is a mineral that, with calcium, makes up most of your bones. Phosphate is obtained through diet, mainly dairy foods. The kidneys usually filter out excess phosphate. If phosphate levels rise too much, it can upset the normal calcium balance of the body. This can lead to thinning of the bones and furring of the arteries.

You may be asked to limit the amount of phosphate in your diet. Foods high in phosphate include red meat, dairy produce, eggs and fish. Your GP or dietitian should be able to advise you about how much phosphate you can eat. However, there is no advantage in reducing your intake of these foods unless you have a raised phosphate level. Always ask a healthcare professional before changing your diet.

If reducing the amount of phosphate in your diet does not lower your phosphate level enough, you may be given medicines called phosphate binders. These medicines bind to the phosphate in the food inside your stomach and stop it from being absorbed into your body.

To work properly, phosphate binders must be taken just before meals. The most commonly used phosphate binder is calcium carbonate, but there are also alternatives that may be more suitable for you.

The side effects of phosphate binders are uncommon but include:

nausea

stomach ache

constipation

diarrhoea

flatulence (wind)

skin rash

itchy skin

Vitamin D supplements

People with kidney disease can have low levels of vitamin D, necessary for healthy bones. This is because the kidneys need to activate the vitamin D from food and the sun before it can be used by the body.

Treatment for kidney failure – transplant or dialysis

Many people with kidney failure can continue with treatment using medicines and will have good-functioning kidneys for the rest of their lives.

In a few people, kidney disease will progress to the stage where the kidneys stop working and it becomes life threatening. This is called kidney failure or established renal failure (ERF).

This rarely happens suddenly, and there will be time to plan the next stage of your condition. The decision whether to have dialysis, a kidney transplant or supportive treatment should be discussed with your healthcare team.

Supportive treatment

If you decide not to have dialysis or a transplant for kidney failure, or they are not suitable for you, you will be offered supportive treatment.

This is also called palliative care.

The aim is to treat and control the symptoms of kidney failure without using dialysis or transplantation. Supportive treatment includes medical, psychological and practical care for both the person with kidney failure and their family, including discussion about how you feel and planning for the end of life.

Many people choose supportive treatment because they:

- are unlikely to benefit or have quality of life with treatment

- do not want to go through the inconvenience of treatment with dialysis

- are advised against dialysis because they have other serious illnesses that will shorten their life, and the negative aspects of treatment outweigh any likely benefits

- have been on dialysis but have decided to stop this treatment

- are being treated with dialysis, but have another serious physical illness, especially severe heart disease or stroke, that will shorten their life

If you choose to have supportive treatment, your kidney unit will still look after you.

Doctors and nurses will make sure you receive:

- medicines to protect your remaining kidney function for as long as possible

- medicines to treat other symptoms of kidney failure, such as feeling out of breath, anaemia, loss of appetite or itchy skin

- help to plan your home and money affairs

- bereavement support for your family after your death

What is good kidney disease care?

According to a national review, kidney disease services should:

- identify people at risk of kidney disease, especially people with high blood pressure or diabetes, and treat them as early as possible to maintain their kidney function

- give people access to investigative treatment and follow them up to reduce the risk of the disease getting worse

- give people good-quality information about managing their condition

- provide information about the development of the disease and treatment options

- provide access to a specialist renal (kidney) team

- give people access to transplant or dialysis services if required

- provide supportive care

Your treatment for kidney disease will need to be reviewed regularly.

It may be helpful for you to make a care plan because this can help you manage your day-to-day health. Your kidney disease specialist nurse may be able to help with this.

Preventing chronic kidney disease

In most cases, chronic kidney disease (CKD) cannot be completely prevented, although you can take steps to reduce the chances of the condition developing.

Managing your condition

If you have a chronic (long-term) condition, such as diabetes, that could potentially cause chronic kidney disease, it is important it is carefully managed.

Follow the advice of your GP and keep all appointments relating to your condition. People with diabetes are advised to have their kidney function tested every year.

Smoking

Smoking increases your risk of cardiovascular disease, including heart attacks or strokes, and it can increase the likelihood that any existing kidney problems will get worse.

If you stop smoking, you will improve your general health and reduce your risk of developing other serious conditions, such as lung cancer and heart disease.

The NHS smoking helpline can offer you advice and encouragement to help you quit smoking. Call Quit Your Way Scotland on 0800 84 84 84.

Diet

A healthy diet is important for preventing chronic kidney disease. It will lower the amount of cholesterol in your blood and keep your blood pressure at a healthy level. Eat a balanced diet that includes plenty of fresh fruit and vegetables (5 A DAY) and whole grains.

Limit the amount of salt in your diet to no more than 6g (0.2oz) a day. Too much salt will increase your blood pressure. One teaspoonful of salt is equal to about 6g.

Avoid eating foods high in saturated fat because this will increase your cholesterol level.

Foods high in saturated fat include:

- meat pies
- sausages and fatty cuts of meat
- butter
- ghee (a type of butter often used in Indian cooking)
- lard
- cream
- hard cheese
- cakes and biscuits

- foods that contain coconut oil or palm oil

Eating some foods that are high in unsaturated fat can help decrease your cholesterol level. Foods high in unsaturated fat include:

- oily fish
- avocados
- nuts and seeds
- sunflower oil
- rapeseed oil
- olive oil

Alcohol

Drinking excessive amounts of alcohol will cause your blood pressure to rise, as well as raising cholesterol levels in your blood. Therefore, sticking to the recommended alcohol consumption limits is the best way to reduce your risk of developing high blood pressure (hypertension) and CKD.

The recommended limits for alcohol are:

- 3-4 units of alcohol a day for men
- 2-3 units of alcohol a day for women

A unit of alcohol is equal to about half a pint of normal strength lager, a small glass of wine or a pub measure (25ml) of spirits.

Exercise

Regular exercise should help lower your blood pressure and reduce your risk of developing CKD.

At least 150 minutes (2 hours and 30 minutes) of moderate-intensity aerobic activity (such as cycling or fast walking) every week, is recommended.

Painkillers

Kidney disease can be caused by the improper use (such as taking too many) of non-steroidal anti-inflammatories (NSAIDs), such as aspirin and ibuprofen.

If you need to take painkillers, make sure you follow the instructions. This can help to avoid kidney damage.

Living with chronic kidney disease

Relationships and support

Coming to terms with a condition such as kidney disease can put a strain on you, your family and your friends. It can be difficult to talk to people about your condition, even if they are close to you.

Learning about kidney disease often helps because you and your family will understand more about what to expect and feel more in control of the illness, instead of feeling that your lives are now dominated by kidney disease and its treatment.

Be open about how you feel, and let your family and friends know what they can do to help. However, do not feel shy about telling them that you need some time to yourself, if that is what you need.

Get support

Your GP or nurse can reassure you if you have questions about your kidney disease, or you may find it helpful to talk to a trained counsellor, psychologist or specialist telephone helpline operator. Your GP surgery will have information on these.

Some people find it helpful to talk to other people with kidney disease at a local support group or through an internet chat room.

Money and finances

If you have to stop work or work part time because of your kidney disease, you may find it hard to cope financially. You may be entitled to one or more of the following types of financial support:

- if you have a job but cannot work because of your illness, you are entitled to Statutory Sick Pay from your employer

- if you do not have a job and cannot work because of your illness, you may be entitled to Employment and Support Allowance

- if you are aged 64 or under and need help with personal care or have walking difficulties, you may be eligible for Disability Living Allowance

- if you are aged 65 or over, you may be able to get Attendance Allowance

- if you are caring for someone with kidney disease, you may be entitled to Carer's Allowance

- you may be eligible for other benefits if you have children living at home or if you have a low household income

National Kidney Federation: Benefits for renal patients and carers

Money Advice Service

Sex and pregnancy

The symptoms of kidney disease and the stress it causes in your life can affect your sexual relationships.

Some couples become closer after a diagnosis of kidney disease, while others find that their loved ones are affected by worries about how they will cope with the effects of the illness. Both men and women may experience issues about body image and self-esteem, and this can affect the relationship.

Try to share your feelings with your partner. If you have problems with sex that do not get better with time, speak to a counsellor or sex therapist.

People on dialysis often experience specific sexual difficulties. Loss of sex drive in both men and women and impotence in men are commonly reported problems.

Treatment is available, but it may take some time and requires commitment from both partners. The first step is to discuss it with your healthcare team.

Pregnancy

Both men and women with early stage kidney disease will find their fertility is unaffected. This means it is important to use contraception unless you want to have a baby.

Later stage kidney disease may affect women's periods, which can make pregnancy more difficult. For men, later stage kidney disease can cause a reduction in sperm count. However, having kidney disease does not mean you will not get pregnant or be able to father a child, so both men and women need to use an effective method of contraception unless they want to have a baby.

Women who want to have a baby should talk to their renal specialist or an obstetrician with an interest in kidney disease. Depending on the stage of kidney disease, there can be risks to both the mother and the baby. It is important to minimise any risk with a planned pregnancy. Your healthcare team can advise you about this.

Holidays and insurance

If you have mild kidney disease or you've had a transplant, going on holiday shouldn't pose additional health problems, whether you're staying in the UK or going abroad.

If you're on dialysis, you can still enjoy holidays provided you book your treatment before you go away.

If you're on dialysis and want to travel, discuss your plans with your renal unit as early as you can. It can sometimes be more difficult to arrange dialysis in the UK than it is abroad.

The NHS will look after you if you get ill while on holiday in the UK. If you're in Europe, the European Health Insurance Card (EHIC) entitles you to free or reduced-cost hospital treatment.

It's a good idea to take out holiday health insurance in addition to carrying the EHIC. Anyone with kidney disease should declare it as a pre-existing medical condition on standard insurance application forms. It may exclude you from some policies.

Using over-the-counter medicines

Some remedies are potentially harmful for people with kidney disease. Make sure you check with your doctor before taking a new over the counter medicine.

You're at higher risk of being harmed by certain over the counter remedies if:

you have advanced kidney disease (stage 4 or 5, or a kidney function below 30% of normal) you have mild-to-moderate kidney disease (stage 3 with a kidney function between 30 and 60% of normal) and are elderly with another serious illness, such as coronary heart disease

What's safe and what's not

Summarised below is a list of which over the counter remedies are safe for people with kidney disease to use and which should be avoided. This is just a guide. For more detailed information, consult your pharmacist, renal specialist or GP.

Headaches

Paracetamol is safe and the best choice of painkiller to treat a headache, but avoid soluble products as they are high in sodium. If your kidney function is less than about 50%, avoid painkillers containing aspirin, ibuprofen or similar drugs such as diclofenac. These products can deteriorate the function of damaged kidneys. Low-dose aspirin of 75-150mg a day can be used if it's prescribed for the prevention of vascular disease. You should also avoid ibuprofen if you're taking anti-rejection treatment following a kidney transplant.

Coughs and colds

Many of the products available for coughs and colds contain a mixture of ingredients, so check the packaging carefully. Some products contain paracetamol, which is safe, but others contain high doses of aspirin, which it's best to avoid.

Many cold remedies also contain decongestants, which you should avoid if you have high blood pressure. The best way to clear congestion is by steam inhalation with menthol or eucalyptus. For coughs, try a simple linctus or glycerine honey and lemon to soothe your throat.

Muscle and joint pains

If you have muscle or joint pain, it's ideal to use topical preparations (applied to the skin), which are rubbed on to the painful area. Avoid tablets containing ibuprofen or similar drugs such as diclofenac if your kidney function is below 50%. Ibuprofen gel or spray is safer than ibuprofen tablets, but it isn't completely risk-free as a small amount of the drug penetrates the skin into the bloodstream.

Kidney failure

About 1% of people with stage three CKD develop kidney failure, also called established renal failure (ERF). Kidney failure has a major impact on your life and the lives of those close to you. People diagnosed with kidney failure usually go through shock, grief and denial before they accept their condition.

Choices if you have established renal failure

If you have established renal failure (ERF), you will need to decide whether to have treatment with dialysis or a kidney transplant. You may decide to have neither treatment and to have supportive care. These choices should be made with your healthcare team.

For people who want active treatment for their ERF, a transplant would be the best option. However, a transplant is only suitable for about half of all people with ERF. This is because they may have had recent cancer or are not physically fit.

Many people who have slowly progressive kidney failure and other serious health problems, and who are usually older, may choose to avoid dialysis. Supportive care can still allow you to live for some time with a good quality of life.

Transplant

A kidney transplant, when suitable, is the best treatment for ERF. The transplanted kidney can be obtained from a deceased or living donor and survival rates are now extremely good. About 90% of transplants still function after five years and many transplants work usefully after 20 years. The main reason people have to wait for a transplant is the shortage of available donors.

Over a third of kidney transplants are now from live donors. A live donor kidney can be transplanted before the need for dialysis, rather than after a period of time on dialysis.

One major risk after transplantation is rejection, where the immune system attacks the donated kidney because it mistakes it for a foreign object. This is prevented with the use of strong drugs to suppress the immune system. These drugs need to be taken meticulously. They are usually well tolerated but may have side effects, including an increased susceptibility to infections and some forms of cancer. For this reason, transplant patients are given regular reviews in a specialist transplant clinic.

Dialysis

Dialysis can take place at home or in hospital. It involves filtering the blood of waste products and excess water. It is not as efficient as a human kidney, so people with kidney failure usually need to restrict their intake of fluid and certain foods. They also require additional medicines such as iron supplements, phosphate binders and antihypertensive medicine (to reduce blood pressure). There are two types of dialysis: peritoneal dialysis and haemodialysis.

Peritoneal dialysis

The abdomen (tummy) has a lining called the peritoneal membrane, which can be used as a filter to remove excess waste and water. If you have opted for peritoneal

76

dialysis, a tube (catheter) will be inserted into your abdomen during an operation. This will allow you to drain dialysis fluid in and out of your tummy yourself. You will not need to go into hospital to be treated, but you will have to spend an hour or two each day draining the fluid. The treatment involves either four exchanges spaced out during the day, each taking half an hour, or attaching yourself to a machine overnight that pumps the fluid in and out for you.

Haemodialysis

Haemodialysis removes waste products and excess fluid that build up in the body when the kidneys stop working. Blood is taken from the body to be cleaned in a filter known as a dialyser. It is effectively an artificial kidney.

77

The whole process takes about four hours and usually has to be repeated three times a week. Most people go into hospital to have haemodialysis. However, some people choose to have the treatment in their own home.

Home haemodialysis will give you more flexibility, but comes with greater responsibility. You'll need to have the space in your home for a dedicated machine and, in most cases, a lot of support from a close family member or friend. Some people choose to have their dialysis at night while they are asleep. Most people who choose home haemodialysis have it every day, so their fluid intake is not as restricted.

Quality vascular access

During haemodialysis, it is important that large volumes of blood are passed through the machine. This requires special measures to get into large enough blood vessels. For this reason, haemodialysis patients need a minor operation to join one of the deep arteries to a superficial vein (called a fistula). This is carried out in day surgery and should be done at least six weeks before dialysis is required because it needs time to mature before it can be used.

Occasionally, there will be insufficient time for a fistula to be created before dialysis is required. In this case, a temporary solution is found, usually involving the use of an indwelling plastic dialysis catheter. A catheter is a surgical tube inserted into the body to allow for the transfer of fluid.

All the issues will be discussed in detail with you by the dialysis team before any decisions are made.

Whole-Foods, Plant-Based Diet: A Detailed Beginner's Guide

There are many arguments about which diet is best for you.

Nevertheless, health and wellness communities agree that diets emphasizing fresh, whole ingredients and minimizing processed foods are superior for overall wellness.

The whole-foods, plant-based diet does just that.

It focuses on minimally processed foods, specifically plants, and is effective at stimulating weight loss and improving health.

This article reviews everything you need to know about the whole-foods, plant-based diet, including its potential health benefits, foods to eat and a sample meal plan.

What Is a Whole-Foods, Plant-Based Diet?

There is no clear definition of a what constitutes a whole-foods, plant-based diet (WFPB diet). The WFPB diet is not necessarily a set diet — it's more of a lifestyle.

This is because plant-based diets can vary greatly depending on the extent to which a person includes animal products in their diet.

Nonetheless, the basic principles of a whole-foods, plant-based diet are as follows:

• Emphasizes whole, minimally processed foods.

• Limits or avoids animal products.

• Focuses on plants, including vegetables, fruits, whole grains, legumes, seeds and nuts, which should make up the majority of what you eat.

• Excludes refined foods, like added sugars, white flour and processed oils.

• Pays special attention to food quality, with many proponents of the WFPB diet promoting locally sourced, organic food whenever possible.

For these reasons, this diet is often confused with vegan or vegetarian diets. Yet although similar in some ways, these diets are not the same.

People who follow vegan diets abstain from consuming any animal products, including dairy, meat, poultry, seafood, eggs and honey. Vegetarians exclude all meat and poultry from their diets, but some vegetarians eat eggs, seafood or dairy.

The WFPB diet, on the other hand, is more flexible. Followers eat mostly plants, but animal products aren't off limits.

While one person following a WFPB diet may eat no animal products, another may eat small amounts of eggs, poultry, seafood, meat or dairy.

SUMMARY

The whole-foods, plant-based diet emphasizes plant-based foods while minimizing animal products and processed items.

It Can Help You Lose Weight and Improve Your Health

Obesity is an issue of epidemic proportions. In fact, over 69% of US adults are overweight or obese.

Fortunately, making dietary and lifestyle changes can facilitate weight loss and have a lasting impact on health.

Many studies have shown that plant-based diets are beneficial for weight loss.

The high fiber content of the WFPB diet, along with the exclusion of processed foods, is a winning combination for shedding excess pounds.

A review of 12 studies that included more than 1,100 people found that those assigned to plant-based diets lost significantly more weight — about 4.5 pounds (2kg) over an average of 18 weeks — than those assigned to non-vegetarian diets.

Adopting a healthy plant-based eating pattern may also help keep weight off in the long run.

A study in 65 overweight and obese adults found that those assigned to a WFPB diet lost significantly more weight than the control group and were able to sustain that weight loss of 9.25 pounds (4.2kg) over a one-year follow-up period.

Plus, simply cutting out the processed foods that aren't allowed on a WFPB diet like soda, candy, fast food and refined grains is a powerful weight loss tool itself.

SUMMARY

Many studies have demonstrated that whole-food, plant-based diets are effective for weight loss. They may also help you maintain weight loss in the long run.

It Benefits a Number of Health

Conditions

Adopting a whole-foods, plant-based diet not only benefits your waistline, but it can also lower your risk and reduce symptoms of certain chronic diseases.

Heart Disease

Perhaps one of the most well-known benefits of WFPB diets is that they are heart-healthy.

However, the quality and types of foods included in the diet matter.

A large study in over 200,000 people found that those who followed a healthy plant-based diet rich in vegetables, fruits, whole-grains, legumes and nuts had a significantly lower risk of developing heart disease than those following non-plant-based diets.

However, unhealthy plant-based diets that included sugary drinks, fruit juices and refined grains were associated with a slightly increased risk of heart disease.

Consuming the right kinds of food is critical for heart disease prevention when following a plant-based diet, which is why adhering to a WFPB diet is the best choice.

Cancer

Research suggests that following a plant-based diet may reduce your risk of certain types of cancer.

A study in over 69,000 people found that vegetarian diets were associated with a significantly lower risk of gastrointestinal cancer, especially for those who followed a lacto-ovo vegetarian diet (vegetarians who eat eggs and dairy.

Another large study in more than 77,000 people demonstrated that those who followed vegetarian diets had a 22% lower risk of developing colorectal cancer than non-vegetarians.

Pescatarians (vegetarians who eat fish) had the greatest protection from colorectal cancer with a 43% reduced risk compared to non-vegetarians.

Cognitive Decline

Some studies suggest that diets rich in vegetables and fruits may help slow or prevent cognitive decline and Alzheimer's disease in older adults.

Plant-based diets have a higher number of plant compounds and antioxidants, which have been shown to slow the progression of Alzheimer's disease and reverse cognitive deficits.

In many studies, higher intakes of fruits and vegetables have been strongly associated with a reduction in cognitive decline.

A review of nine studies including over 31,000 people found that eating more fruits and vegetables led to a 20% reduction in the risk of developing cognitive impairment or dementia.

Diabetes

Adopting a WFPB diet may be an effective tool in managing and reducing your risk of developing diabetes.

A study in more than 200,000 people found that those who adhered to a healthy plant-based eating pattern had a 34% lower risk of developing diabetes than those who followed unhealthy, non-plant-based diets.

Another study demonstrated that plant-based diets (vegan and lacto-ovo vegetarian) were associated with nearly a 50% reduction in the risk of type 2 diabetes compared to non-vegetarian diets.

Plus, plant-based diets have been shown to improve blood sugar control in people with diabetes.

SUMMARY

Following a whole-foods, plant-based diet may reduce your risk of developing heart disease, certain cancers, cognitive decline and diabetes.

Adopting a Whole-Foods, Plant-Based Diet Is Good for the Planet

Switching to a plant-based diet not only benefits your health — it can help protect the environment, as well.

People who follow plant-based diets tend to have smaller environmental footprints.

Adopting sustainable eating habits can help reduce greenhouse gas emissions, water consumption and land used for factory farming, which are all factors in global warming and environmental degradation.

A review of 63 studies showed that the largest environmental benefits were seen from diets containing the least amount of animal-based foods such as vegan, vegetarian and pescatarian diets.

The study reported that a 70% reduction in greenhouse gas emissions and land use and 50% less water use could be achieved by shifting Western diet patterns to more sustainable, plant-based dietary patterns.

What's more, reducing the number of animal products in your diet and purchasing local, sustainable produce helps drive the local economy and reduces reliance on factory farming, an unsustainable method of food production.

SUMMARY

Plant-based diets emphasizing local ingredients are more environmentally friendly than diets that rely heavily on mass-produced animal products and produce.

Foods to Eat on a Whole-Foods, Plant-Based Diet

From eggs and bacon for breakfast to steak for dinner, animal products are the focus of most meals for many people.

When switching to a plant-based diet, meals should center around plant-based foods.

If animal foods are eaten, they should be eaten in smaller quantities, with attention paid to the quality of the item.

Foods like dairy, eggs, poultry, meat and seafood should be used more as a complement to a plant-based meal, not as the main focal point.

A Whole-Foods, Plant-Based Shopping List

• Fruits: Berries, citrus fruits, pears, peaches, pineapple, bananas, etc.

• Vegetables: Kale, spinach, tomatoes, broccoli, cauliflower, carrots, asparagus, peppers, etc.

• Starchy vegetables: Potatoes, sweet potatoes, butternut squash, etc.

- Whole grains: Brown rice, rolled oats, farro, quinoa, brown rice pasta, barley, etc.

- Healthy fats: Avocados, olive oil, coconut oil, unsweetened coconut, etc.

- Legumes: Peas, chickpeas, lentils, peanuts, black beans, etc.

- Seeds, nuts and nut butters: Almonds, cashews, macadamia nuts, pumpkin seeds, sunflower seeds, natural peanut butter, tahini, etc.

- Unsweetened plant-based milks: Coconut milk, almond milk, cashew milk, etc.

- Spices, herbs and seasonings: Basil, rosemary, turmeric, curry, black pepper, salt, etc.

- Condiments: Salsa, mustard, nutritional yeast, soy sauce, vinegar, lemon juice, etc.

• Plant-based protein: Tofu, tempeh, plant-based protein sources or powders with no added sugar or artificial ingredients.

• Beverages: Coffee, tea, sparkling water, etc.

If supplementing your plant-based diet with animal products, choose quality products from grocery stores or, better yet, purchase them from local farms.

• Eggs: Pasture-raised when possible.

• Poultry: Free-range, organic when possible.

• Beef and pork: Pastured or grass-fed when possible.

• Seafood: Wild-caught from sustainable fisheries when possible.

• Dairy: Organic dairy products from pasture-raised animals whenever possible.

SUMMARY

A healthy, WFPB diet should focus on plant foods like vegetables, fruits, whole grains, legumes, nuts and seeds. If animal products are eaten, they should be eaten in smaller quantities compared to plant foods.

Foods to Avoid or Minimize on This Diet

The WFPB diet is a way of eating that focuses on consuming foods in their most natural form. This means that heavily processed foods are excluded.

When purchasing groceries, focus on fresh foods and, when purchasing foods with a label, aim for items with the fewest possible ingredients.

Foods to Avoid

- Fast food: French fries, cheeseburgers, hot dogs, chicken nuggets, etc.

- Added sugars and sweets: Table sugar, soda, juice, pastries, cookies, candy, sweet tea, sugary cereals, etc.

- Refined grains: White rice, white pasta, white bread, bagels, etc.

- Packaged and convenience foods: Chips, crackers, cereal bars, frozen dinners, etc.

- Processed vegan-friendly foods: Plant-based meats like Tofurkey, faux cheeses, vegan butters, etc.

- Artificial sweeteners: Equal, Splenda, Sweet'N Low, etc.

- Processed animal products: Bacon, lunch meats, sausage, beef jerky, etc.

Foods to Minimize

While healthy animal foods can be included in a WFPB diet, the following products should be minimized in all plant-based diets.

- Beef

- Pork

- Sheep

- Game meats

- Poultry

- Eggs

- Dairy

- Seafood

SUMMARY

When following a WFPB diet, highly processed foods should be avoided and animal products minimized.

A Sample Meal Plan for One Week

Transitioning to a whole-foods, plant-based diet doesn't have to be challenging.

The following one-week menu can help set you up for success. It includes a small number of animal products, but the extent to which you include animal foods in your diet is up to you.

Monday

• Breakfast: Oatmeal made with coconut milk topped with berries, coconut and walnuts.

- Lunch: Large salad topped with fresh vegetables, chickpeas, avocado, pumpkin seeds and goat cheese.

- Dinner: Butternut squash curry.

Tuesday

- Breakfast: Full-fat plain yogurt topped with sliced strawberries, unsweetened coconut and pumpkin seeds.

- Lunch: Meatless chili.

- Dinner: Sweet potato and black bean tacos.

Wednesday

- Breakfast: A smoothie made with unsweetened coconut milk, berries, peanut butter and unsweetened plant-based protein powder.

- Lunch: Hummus and veggie wrap.

• Dinner: Zucchini noodles tossed in pesto with chicken meatballs.

Thursday

• Breakfast: Savory oatmeal with avocado, salsa and black beans.

• Lunch: Quinoa, veggie and feta salad.

• Dinner: Grilled fish with roasted sweet potatoes and broccoli.

Friday

• Breakfast: Tofu and vegetable frittata.

• Lunch: Large salad topped with grilled shrimp.

• Dinner: Roasted portobello fajitas.

Saturday

• Breakfast: Blackberry, kale, cashew butter and coconut protein smoothie.

• Lunch: Vegetable, avocado and brown rice sushi with a seaweed salad.

• Dinner: Eggplant lasagna made with cheese and a large green salad.

Sunday

• Breakfast: Vegetable omelet made with eggs.

• Lunch: Roasted vegetable and tahini quinoa bowl.

• Dinner: Black bean burgers served on a large salad with sliced avocado.

As you can see, the idea of a whole-foods, plant-based diet is to use animal products sparingly.

However, many people following WFPB diets eat more or fewer animal products depending on their specific dietary needs and preferences.

SUMMARY

You can enjoy many different delicious meals when following a whole-foods, plant-based diet. The above menu can help you get started.

The Bottom Line

A whole-foods, plant-based diet is a way of eating that celebrates plant foods and cuts out unhealthy items like added sugars and refined grains.

Plant-based diets have been linked to a number of health benefits, including reducing your risk of heart disease, certain cancers, obesity, diabetes and cognitive decline.

Plus, transitioning to a more plant-based diet is an excellent choice for the planet.

Regardless of the type of whole-foods, plant-based diet you choose, adopting this way of eating is sure to boost your health.

The 7 Best Plant Sources of Omega-3 Fatty Acids

Omega-3 fatty acids are important fats that provide many health benefits.

Studies have found that they may reduce inflammation, decrease blood triglycerides and even reduce the risk of dementia.

The most well-known sources of omega-3 fatty acids include fish oil and fatty fish like salmon, trout and tuna.

This can make it challenging for vegans, vegetarians or even those who simply dislike fish to meet their omega-3 fatty acid needs.

Of the three main types of omega-3 fatty acids, plant foods typically only contain alpha-linolenic acid (ALA).

ALA is not as active in the body and must be converted to two other forms of omega-3 fatty acids — eicosapentaenoic acid (EPA) and docosahexaenoic acid (DHA) — to bestow the same health benefits.

Unfortunately, your body's ability to convert ALA is limited. Only about 5% of ALA is converted to EPA, while less than 0.5% is converted to DHA.

Thus, if you don't supplement with fish oil or get EPA or DHA from your diet, it's important to eat a good amount of ALA-rich foods to meet your omega-3 needs.

Additionally, keep in mind your omega-6 to omega-3 ratio, as a diet low in omega-3s but high in omega-6s can increase inflammation and your risk of disease.

Here are 7 of the best plant sources of omega-3 fatty acids.

Chia Seeds

Chia seeds are known for their many health benefits, bringing a hefty dose of fiber and protein with each serving.

They're also a great plant-based source of ALA omega-3 fatty acids.

Thanks to their omega-3, fiber and protein, studies have found chia seeds could decrease the risk of chronic disease when consumed as part of a healthy diet.

One study found that consuming a diet with chia seeds, nopal, soy protein and oats decreased blood triglycerides, glucose intolerance and inflammatory markers.

A 2007 animal study also found that eating chia seeds decreased blood triglycerides and increased both "good" HDL cholesterol and omega-3 levels in the blood.

Just one ounce (28 grams) of chia seeds can meet and exceed your daily recommended intake of omega-3 fatty acids, delivering a whopping 4,915 mg (9).

The current daily recommended intake of ALA for adults over age 19 is 1,100 mg for women and 1,600 mg for men (10).

Boost your chia seed intake by whipping up a nutritious chia pudding or sprinkle chia seeds on top of salads, yogurts or smoothies.

Ground chia seeds can also be used as a vegan substitute for eggs. Combine one tablespoon (7 grams) with 3 tablespoons of water to replace one egg in recipes.

SUMMARY:

One ounce (28 grams) of chia seeds provides 4,915 mg of ALA omega-3 fatty acids, meeting 307–447% of the recommended daily intake.

Brussels Sprouts

In addition to their high content of vitamin K, vitamin C and fiber, Brussels sprouts are an excellent source of omega-3 fatty acids.

Because cruciferous vegetables like Brussels sprouts are so rich in nutrients and omega-3 fatty acids, they have been linked to many health benefits.

In fact, one study found that an increased intake of cruciferous vegetables is associated with a 16% lower risk of heart disease.

A half cup (44 grams) of raw Brussels sprouts contains about 44 mg of ALA (12).

Meanwhile, cooked Brussels sprouts contain three times as much, providing 135 mg of omega-3 fatty acids in each half-cup (78-gram) serving (13).

Whether they're roasted, steamed, blanched or stir-fried, Brussels sprouts make a healthy and delicious accompaniment to any meal.

SUMMARY:

Each half-cup (78-gram) serving of cooked Brussels sprouts contains 135 mg of ALA, or up to 12% of the daily recommended intake.

Algal Oil

Algal oil, a type of oil derived from algae, stands out as one of the few vegan sources of both EPA and DHA.

Some studies have even found that it's comparable to seafood in regard to its nutritional availability of EPA and DHA.

One study compared algal oil capsules to cooked salmon and found that both were well tolerated and equivalent in terms of absorption.

Though research is limited, animal studies show that the DHA from algal oil is especially beneficial to health.

In fact, a recent animal study found that supplementing mice with a DHA algal oil compound led to an improvement in memory.

However, more studies are needed to determine the extent of its health benefits.

Most commonly available in softgel form, algal oil supplements typically provide 400–500 mg of combined DHA and EPA. Generally, it is recommended to get 300–900 mg of combined DHA and EPA per day.

Algal oil supplements are easy to find in most pharmacies. Liquid forms can also be added to drinks or smoothies for a dose of healthy fats.

SUMMARY:

Depending on the supplement, algal oil provides 400–500 mg of DHA and EPA, fulfilling 44–167% of the daily recommended intake.

Hemp Seed

In addition to protein, magnesium, iron and zinc, hemp seeds are comprised of about 30% oil and contain a good amount of omega-3s.

Animal studies have found that the omega-3s found in hemp seeds could benefit heart health.

They may do this by preventing the formation of blood clots and helping the heart recover after a heart attack.

Each ounce (28 grams) of hemp seeds contains approximately 6,000 mg of ALA (22Trusted Source).

Sprinkle hemp seeds on top of yogurt or mix them into a smoothie to add a bit of crunch and boost the omega-3 content of your snack.

Also, homemade hemp seed granola bars can be a simple way to combine hemp seeds with other healthy ingredients like flaxseeds and pack in extra omega-3s.

Hemp seed oil, which is made by pressing hemp seeds, can also be consumed to provide a concentrated dose of omega-3 fatty acids.

SUMMARY:

One ounce (28 grams) of hemp seeds contains 6,000 mg of ALA omega-3 fatty acids, or 375–545% of the daily recommended intake.

Walnuts

Walnuts are loaded with healthy fats and ALA omega-3 fatty acids. In fact, walnuts are comprised of about 65% fat by weight.

Several animal studies have found that walnuts could help improve brain health due to their omega-3 content.

A 2011 animal study found that eating walnuts was associated with improvements in learning and memory.

Another animal study showed walnuts caused significant improvements in memory, learning, motor development and anxiety in mice with Alzheimer's disease.

Just one serving of walnuts can fulfill an entire day's requirements of omega-3 fatty acids, with a single ounce (28 grams) providing 2,542 mg (26).

Add walnuts to your homemade granola or cereal, sprinkle them on top of yogurt or simply snack on a handful to increase your ALA intake.

SUMMARY:

One ounce (28 grams) of walnuts contains 2,542 mg of ALA omega-3 fatty acids, or 159–231% of the daily recommended intake.

Flaxseeds

Flaxseeds are nutritional powerhouses, providing a good amount of fiber, protein, magnesium and manganese in each serving.

They're also an excellent source of omega-3s.

Several studies have demonstrated the heart-healthy benefits of flaxseeds, largely thanks to their omega-3 fatty acid content.

Both flaxseeds and flaxseed oil have been shown to reduce cholesterol in multiple studies.

Another study found that flaxseeds could help significantly lower blood pressure, particularly in those with high blood pressure.

One ounce (28 grams) of flaxseeds contains 6,388 mg of ALA omega-3 fatty acids, surpassing the daily recommended amount (31).

Flaxseeds are easy to incorporate into your diet and can be a staple ingredient in vegan baking.

Whisk together one tablespoon (7 grams) of flaxseed meal with 2.5 tablespoons of water to use it as a handy substitute for one egg in baked goods.

With a mild yet slightly nutty flavor, flaxseed also makes the perfect addition to cereal, oatmeal, soups or salads.

SUMMARY:

One ounce (28 grams) of flaxseeds contains 6,388 mg of ALA omega-3 fatty acids, or 400–580% of the daily recommended intake.

Perilla Oil

This oil, derived from perilla seeds, is often used in Korean cuisine as a condiment and cooking oil.

In addition to being a versatile and flavorful ingredient, it's also a good source of omega-3 fatty acids.

One study in 20 elderly participants replaced soybean oil with perilla oil and found that it caused ALA levels in the blood to double. In the long term, it also led to an increase in EPA and DHA blood levels.

Perilla oil is very rich in omega-3 fatty acids, with ALA making up an estimated 64% of this seed oil.

Each tablespoon (14 grams) contains nearly 9,000 mg of ALA omega-3 fatty acids.

To maximize its health benefits, perilla oil should be used as a flavor enhancer or dressing, rather than a cooking oil. This is because oils high in polyunsaturated fats can oxidize with heat, forming harmful free radicals that contribute to disease.

Perilla oil is also available in capsule form for an easy and convenient way to increase your omega-3 intake.

SUMMARY:

Each tablespoon (14 grams) of perilla oil contains 9,000 mg of ALA omega-3 fatty acids, or 563–818% of the daily recommended intake.

The Bottom Line

Omega-3 fatty acids are an important part of the diet and essential to your health.

If you don't eat fish because of dietary reasons or personal preference, you can still reap the benefits of omega-3 fatty acids in your diet.

By either incorporating a few omega-3-rich foods into your diet or opting for a plant-based supplement, it's possible to meet your needs, seafood-free.

What Is Escarole, and How Is It Eaten?

If you enjoy Italian food, you might have already encountered escarole — a leafy, bitter green that looks a lot like lettuce.

Escarole is a traditional ingredient in Italian wedding soup, which usually combines this vegetable with a small, round pasta and meatballs or sausage in chicken broth. This hearty green can also be found in stews, salads, and pastas.

However, many people don't know whether to classify escarole as an endive or a lettuce.

This article explains all you need to know about escarole, including its nutrients, health benefits, and culinary uses.

What is escarole?

Escarole (Cichorium endivia) is a member of the chicory family. It's often confused not only with lettuce but also its botanical relatives, which include curly endive, radicchio, frisée, and other bitter green vegetables (1, 2).

Technically, escarole is considered a flat-leafed variety of endive. What's commonly called "endive" is Belgian endive, a yellow-green plant with tightly layered, cylindrical leaves (2).

All the same, you'll usually find this hearty plant bunched in with the kales and lettuces at the supermarket.

While escarole looks a lot like butterhead lettuce, you can tell them apart because escarole has wide, green leaves with slightly jagged, crumpled edges that cluster into a rosette — whereas the broad leaves of lettuce are wavy and smooth (1, 2).

Unlike lettuce, escarole offers a pleasant bitterness and versatility. It's milder and tenderer than curly endive.

While native to the East Indies, escarole grows in a variety of climates and is now found across the globe. It's especially popular in Italian cuisine (2).

SUMMARY

Escarole is a flat-leafed endive that belongs to the chicory family. Its broad leaves have crumpled, slightly jagged edges that distinguish it from butterhead lettuce. While bitterer than lettuce, it's less sharp than curly endive.

Nutritional profile

Like other members of the chicory family, escarole gets its bitter notes from a plant compound called lactucopicrin, which is also known as intybin (3, 4).

Plus, similarly to other leafy greens, this veggie packs amble nutrients into very few calories. Every 2 cups (85 grams) of raw escarole — about one-sixth of a medium head — provides (5, 6):

- Calories: 15

- Carbs: 3 grams

- Protein: 1 gram

- Fat: 0 grams

- Fiber: 3 grams

- Iron: 4% of the Daily Value (DV)

- Vitamin A: 58% of the DV

- Vitamin K: 164% of the DV

- Vitamin C: 10% of the DV

- Folate: 30% of the DV

- Zinc: 6% of the DV

- Copper: 9% of the DV

With very few calories and no fat, escarole heaps micronutrients and fiber — just 2 raw cups (85 grams) deliver 12% of the DV for fiber (7).

What's more, this same serving provides 9% of the DV for copper and 30% for folate. Copper supports proper bone, connective tissue, and red blood cell formation, whereas folate helps ensure proper metabolism and create red and white blood cells (8, 9).

Both minerals are especially important for proper fetal development and thus vital for women who are pregnant or planning to become pregnant (9, 10).

SUMMARY

Escarole packs fiber and several nutrients, including copper, folate, and vitamins A, C, and K — all with very few calories and zero fat.

Health benefits of escarole

Escarole is nutrient-dense and boasts many potential health benefits.

May promote gut health

The two types of fiber — soluble and insoluble — act differently in your body.

While soluble fiber bulks up your stool and feeds the friendly bacteria in your gut, the insoluble type passes through your digestive system unchanged, promoting gut health by pushing food through your gut and stimulating bowel movements (7).

Notably, escarole provides mostly insoluble fiber. Boasting 12% of your daily fiber needs per 2 cups (85 gram), it can help keep your bowels regular and prevent the discomfort of constipation and piles (5, 6, 7).

May support eye health

Escarole is rich in provitamin A, providing 54% of the DV in only 2 cups (85 grams) (5, 6).

This vitamin promotes eye health, as it's an important component of rhodopsin, a pigment in your retina that helps discern between lightness and darkness.

Chronic vitamin A deficiencies are linked to visual issues like night blindness, a condition in which people can't see well at night but have no trouble with their vision in the daylight.

Vitamin A deficiencies are also associated with macular degeneration, an age-related decline in eyesight that results in blindness.

May reduce inflammation

In addition to its impressive nutrient profile, escarole boasts many powerful antioxidants, which are compounds that defend your body against oxidative stress and unstable molecules called free radicals. Long-term oxidative stress may trigger inflammation (13).

Studies suggest that kaempferol, an antioxidant in escarole, may safeguard your cells against chronic inflammation.

Yet, these studies are limited to rats and test tubes. Human research is needed to fully understand kaempferol's effects on inflammation.

May promote bone and heart health

Vitamin K is important for normal blood clotting, as well as regulating calcium levels in your heart and bones. Leafy greens like escarole deliver a subtype called vitamin K1.

This vegetable offers a whopping 164% of your daily needs of this nutrient per 2-cup (85-gram) raw serving.

A 2-year study in 440 postmenopausal women found that supplementing with 5 mg of vitamin K1 daily resulted in a 50% reduction in bone fractures, compared with a placebo group (18Trusted Source).

Furthermore, a 3-year study in 181 postmenopausal women found that combining vitamin K1 with vitamin D significantly slowed the hardening of arteries associated with heart disease (18Trusted Source).

Sufficient vitamin K intake is associated with a decreased risk of heart disease and early death from this condition (18Trusted Source).

SUMMARY

Escarole's many benefits include supporting gut and eye health. It may likewise reduce inflammation and promote proper blood clotting and bone health.

How to prepare and eat escarole

Escarole is a versatile veggie but lends itself particularly well to raw salads and heartier dishes. Its outer leaves are bitter and chewy, while its yellow inner leaves are sweeter and tenderer.

An acid like lemon juice or vinegar counters the bitterness of raw escarole. If you're sensitive to sharp flavors, cooking it will also help mellow it out. In this vein, you can sauté it or add it to a soup.

Escarole even works on the grill. To grill it, cut the vegetable into fourths lengthwise. Then, brush on canola oil, which has a higher smoke point than most other oils and is less likely to generate toxic compounds at high heat (19, 20).

Then sprinkle on salt and pepper and grill it for about 3 minutes per side. Serve it with your favorite sauces or dips, such as a lemony Greek yogurt or white bean dip.

SUMMARY

You can eat escarole raw in salads or cook it in a variety of ways, including sautéing and grilling. Adding acids will tone down its bitterness, as will cooking it.

Precautions

Like any raw vegetable, escarole should be thoroughly washed in clean, running water before eating it. This reduces the threat of foodborne illnesses by flushing out harmful bacteria (21, 22).

Though this leafy green is incredibly healthy, people who take blood thinners may want to moderate their intake.

That's because blood thinners like warfarin are known to interact with vitamin K. Rapid fluctuations in levels of this vitamin can counter the effects of your blood thinner, putting you at risk of serious side effects, such as blood clots, which can lead to stroke and heart attack (23, 24).

What's more, eating escarole regularly can exacerbate kidney stones in people with kidney problems. Its high content of oxalate — a plant compound that helps get rid of excess calcium — may be to blame, as this substance is filtered by your kidneys (25).

SUMMARY

Be sure to wash your escarole thoroughly before eating it. People who take blood thinners or have kidney problems may also want to monitor their intake.

The bottom line

Escarole is a broad-leafed endive that looks like butterhead lettuce save for its slightly crumpled, jagged leaves. To balance out its bitter notes, you can cook it or sprinkle on lemon juice or vinegar.

This vegetable boasts numerous benefits for your eyes, guts, bones, and heart. It makes a great addition to salads and soups — and can even be grilled.

If you're interested in varying up your veggie routine, give this unique leafy green a try.

21 Reasons to Eat Real Food

Real food is whole, single-ingredient food.

It is mostly unprocessed, free of chemical additives, and rich in nutrients.

In essence, it's the type of food human beings ate exclusively for thousands of years.

However, since processed foods became popular in the 20th century, the Western diet has shifted toward ready-to-eat meals.

While processed foods are convenient, they also harm your health. In fact, following a diet based on real food may be one of the most important things you can do to maintain good health and a high quality of life.

Here are 21 reasons to eat real food.

1. Loaded with important nutrients

Unprocessed animal and plant foods provide the vitamins and minerals you need for optimal health.

For instance, 1 cup (220 grams) of red bell peppers, broccoli, or orange slices contains more than 100% of the RDI for vitamin C.

Eggs and liver are especially high in choline, a nutrient essential for proper brain function.

And a single Brazil nut provides all the selenium you need for an entire day (6).

In fact, most whole foods are good sources of vitamins, minerals, and other beneficial nutrients.

2. Low in sugar

Some research suggests that eating sugary foods can increase your risk of obesity, insulin resistance, type 2 diabetes, fatty liver disease, and heart disease.

Generally speaking, real food is lower in sugar than many processed foods.

Even though fruit contains sugar, it's also high in water and fiber, making it much healthier than soda and processed foods.

3. Heart healthy

Real food is packed with antioxidants and nutrients that support heart health, including magnesium and healthy fats.

Eating a diet rich in nutritious, unprocessed foods may also help reduce inflammation, which is considered one of the major drivers of heart disease (10).

4. Better for the environment

The world population is steadily growing, and with this growth comes increased demand for food.

However, producing food for billions of people has an environmental toll.

This is partly due to the destruction of rainforests for agricultural land, increased fuel needs, pesticide use, greenhouse gases, and packaging that ends up in landfills.

Developing sustainable agriculture based on real food may help improve the health of the planet by reducing energy needs and decreasing the amount of non-biodegradable waste that humans produce.

5. High in fiber

Fiber provides many health benefits, including boosting digestive function, metabolic health, and feelings of fullness.

Foods like avocados, chia seeds, flaxseeds, and blackberries are particularly high in healthy fiber, alongside beans and legumes.

Consuming fiber through whole foods is much better than taking a supplement or eating processed food with added fiber.

6. Helps control blood sugar

According to the International Diabetes Federation, more than 400 million people have diabetes worldwide.

That number is expected to surpass 600 million within the next 25 years.

Eating a diet high in fibrous plants and unprocessed animal foods may help reduce blood sugar levels in people who have or are at risk for diabetes.

In one 12-week study, people with diabetes or prediabetes followed a paleolithic diet combining fresh meat, fish, fruits, vegetables, eggs, and nuts. They experienced a 26% reduction in blood sugar levels.

7. Good for your skin

In addition to promoting better overall health, real food nourishes and helps protect your skin.

For instance, dark chocolate and avocados have been shown to protect skin against sun damage.

Studies suggest that eating more vegetables, fish, beans, and olive oil may help reduce wrinkling, loss of elasticity, and other age-related skin changes.

What's more, switching from a Western diet high in processed foods to one based on real food may help prevent or reduce acne (20Trusted Source).

8. Helps lower triglycerides

Blood triglyceride levels are strongly influenced by food intake.

Because triglycerides tend to go up when you eat sugar and refined carbs, it's best to minimize these foods or cut them out of your diet altogether.

In addition, including unprocessed foods like fatty fish, lean meats, vegetables, and nuts has been shown to significantly reduce triglyceride levels.

9. Provides variety

Eating the same foods over and over can get old. It's healthier to include diverse foods in your diet.

Hundreds of different real food options exist, including a wide variety of meat, fish, dairy, vegetables, fruits, nuts, legumes, whole grains, and seeds.

Make a point of regularly trying new foods. Some unique options include chayote squash, chia seeds, organ meats, kefir, and quinoa.

10. Costs less in the long run

It's said that real food is more expensive than processed food.

In some ways, this adage holds true. An analysis of 27 studies from 10 countries found that eating healthier food costs about $1.56 more than processed food per 2,000 calories (23).

However, this difference is minimal compared to the cost of managing chronic lifestyle diseases, such as diabetes and obesity.

For instance, one study noted that people with diabetes spend 2.3 times more on medical supplies and health care than those who don't have this condition (24Trusted Source).

Thus, real food costs less in the long run because it's more likely to keep you healthy, minimizing your medical costs.

11. High in healthy fats

Unlike the trans and processed fats found in vegetable oils and spreads, most naturally occurring fats are healthy.

For example, extra virgin olive oil is a great source of oleic acid, a monounsaturated fat that promotes heart health (25Trusted Source).

Coconut oil contains medium-chain triglycerides, which may increase fat burning and assist with weight loss.

What's more, long-chain omega-3 fatty acids help fight inflammation and protect heart health. Fatty fish, such as salmon, herring and sardines, are excellent sources.

Other real foods that are high in healthy fats include avocados, nuts, seeds, and whole-milk dairy.

12. May reduce disease risk

Making real food part of your lifestyle may help reduce your risk of disease.

Eating patterns — like the Mediterranean diet — based on whole, unprocessed foods have been shown to reduce your risk of heart disease, diabetes, and metabolic syndrome.

In addition, several large observational studies link a balanced diet heavy in fruits and vegetables to a decreased risk of cancer and heart disease.

13. Contains antioxidants

Antioxidants are compounds that help fight free radicals, which are unstable molecules that can damage your body's cells.

They are found in all real foods, especially plant foods like vegetables, fruits, nuts, whole grains, and legumes. Fresh, unprocessed animal foods also contain antioxidants — though in much lower levels.

For instance, egg yolks offer lutein and zeaxanthin, which help protect against eye diseases like cataracts and macular degeneration (34Trusted Source, 35Trusted Source).

14. Good for your gut

Eating real food may be beneficial for your gut microbiome, which refers to the bacteria that live in your digestive tract.

Indeed, many real foods function as prebiotics — food that your gut bacteria ferment into short-chain fatty acids. In addition to promoting gut health, these fatty acids may improve blood sugar control.

Real food sources of prebiotics include garlic, asparagus, and cocoa.

15. May help prevent overeating

A high intake of processed and fast foods has been linked to overeating, particularly in those who are overweight.

By contrast, real food doesn't harbor the sugars and flavorings that load down processed foods and may drive overeating.

16. Promotes dental health

Healthy teeth may be another benefit of real foods.

The sugar and refined carbs in the Western diet promote dental decay by feeding the plaque-causing bacteria that live in your mouth. The combination of sugar and acid in soda is especially likely to cause decay.

Cheese seems to help prevent cavities by increasing pH and hardening tooth enamel. One study found that eating cheese dramatically improved enamel strength in people with limited saliva production.

Green tea has also been shown to protect tooth enamel. One study found rinsing with green tea significantly reduced the amount of erosion that occurred when people drank soda and brushed their teeth vigorously (41Trusted Source).

17. May help reduce sugar cravings

A diet based on real food may also help reduce cravings for sweets like cakes, cookies, and candy.

Once your body adjusts to eating whole, unprocessed foods, cravings for sugary foods could become infrequent and even disappear altogether. Your taste buds eventually adapt to appreciate real food.

18. Sets a good example

In addition to improving your own health and well-being, eating real food can help the people you care about stay healthy.

Leading by example can encourage your friends and family to adopt better eating habits. It's also a good way to help your kids learn about good nutrition.

19. Gets the focus off dieting

A dieting mentality may be harmful because it limits your focus to your weight.

In fact, good nutrition is about much more than losing weight. It's also about having enough energy and feeling healthy.

Focusing on real food instead of dieting can be a much more sustainable and enjoyable way to live. Instead of forcing weight loss, let weight loss come as a natural side effect of a better diet and improved metabolic health.

20. Helps support local farmers

Purchasing produce, meat, and dairy from farmers markets supports the people who grow food in your community.

In addition, local farms often provide much fresher and less processed food than supermarkets.

21. Delicious

On top of everything else, real food tastes delicious.

The amazing flavor of fresh, unprocessed food is undeniable.

Once your taste buds have adjusted to real food, processed junk food simply can't compare.

The bottom line

Real food is just one component of a healthy lifestyle.

It's also important to get plenty of exercise, lower your stress levels, and maintain proper nutrition.

But there's no doubt that eating more real food will go a long way toward improving your health.

Baked Ikarian Chickpeas

Ikarians eat a variation of the Mediterranean diet, with lots of fruits and vegetables, whole grains, beans, potatoes and olive oil. Olive oil contains cholesterol-lowering mono-unsaturated fats.

Try this delicious Baked Chickpeas recipe. And don't forget the olive oil!

INGREDIENTS

- 1 pound dried chickpeas

- 1 zucchini cut into ½ inch cubes

- 2 carrots cut into ½ inch cubes

- 1 small onion cut into ½ inch cubes

• Mint leaves (dried or fresh)

• Olive Oil

DIRECTIONS

1. Soak chickpeas.

2. With fresh water, bring peas to a boil for 5 mins.

3. Drain off water and rinse chickpeas with fresh water, and bring back to a boil. Cook until almost done (firm, not hard)

4. Mix vegetables together with mint and toss liberally with olive oil. Then spread out in the bottom of a large baking pan.

5. Add cooked chickpeas on top and about a ¼ inch of chickpea water to vegetables.

6. Bake in a preheated over at 350 degrees for about 15 minutes or until vegetables and chickpeas are tender (chickpeas should be slightly browned.)

7. Toss, salt and pepper to taste.

Ikarian Tabouli Salad

Ikaria's traditional diet, like that found in much of the Mediterranean, includes a lot of vegetables and olive oil, small amounts of dairy and meat products, and moderate amounts of alcohol. Its emphasis on legumes, wild greens and olive oil contribute to the island's extreme longevity. Tabouli is a traditional Mediterranean dish that features parsley as the star of the show. The secret to a traditional Ikarian tabouli is the ratio of bulgar to parsley. Be sure you have a tabouli salad with a little bit of bulgar, not a bowl of bulgar with a little bit of salad.

INGREDIENTS

- 1/3 cup bulgur wheat, rinsed

- 5 bunches parsley, finely chopped

- 5 medium tomatoes, diced small

- 1/2 cup chopped green onions

- 3 lemons, freshly squeezed

- 1/4 cup mint

- 1/2 cup extra-virgin olive oil

- 1/2 tbsp salt, or to taste

- 1/2 tsp pepper, or to taste

DIRECTIONS

1. Mix all ingredients together and enjoy.

Note: This also makes a great leftover salad.

Yield: Serves 8

Per serving: 144 calories, 13.5g fat, 151mg sodium, 1g fiber, 1g protein

Savory Roasted Chickpeas

Move over croutons, chickpeas are the new salad topper! Roasting your chickpeas will bring a whole new taste and appeal to this little bean. Toss them onto a salad or package them up for an afternoon snack.

INGREDIENTS

- 1- 15 ounce can chickpeas, rinsed and drained

- 2 Tablespoons olive oil

- 1 teaspoon ground cumin

- 2 teaspoons chili powder

- 1 teaspoon cayenne pepper

- 1 teaspoon sea salt

DIRECTIONS

1. Preheat oven to 400 degrees. Drain and rinse the chickpeas.

2. Lie out a clean kitchen towel or several layers of paper towels and lay the chickpeas over the top. Gently dry the chickpeas in the towels until they are very dry.

3. In a large bowl, combine the oils and spices. Add the chickpeas to the bowl and toss until evenly coated.

4. Pour the chickpeas in an even layer onto a sheet pan with sides lined with foil.

5. Bake for 35-45 minutes, stirring every 10 minutes until crispy and golden brown.

Serves 4

Sweet Roasted Chickpeas

DESSERT / SNACK

Savory roasted chickpeas are great for a salty snack or salad topping, but what about when you're craving something sweet? These sweet roasted chickpeas with kill your craving with a hint of sweetness and natural maple syrup.

INGREDIENTS

- 1 15-oz can chickpeas, rinsed and drained

- 1-2 tsp coconut oil

- 1-2 tsp ground cinnamon

- 1-2 tsp sugar or coconut sugar

- 1/2 tsp cayenne pepper

- 1 tbsp maple syrup or honey

- pinch of salt

DIRECTIONS

1. Preheat oven to 400 degrees.

2. Drain and rinse chickpeas well. Lie out a clean kitchen towel or several layers of paper towels and pour the chickpeas out. Gently pat chickpeas until they are very dry.

3. In a large bowl, combine the oil and spices. Add the chickpeas to the bowl and toss until evenly coated.

4. Pour the chickpeas in an even layer onto a sheet pan with sides lined with foil.

5. Bake for 25-30 minutes, stirring every 10 minutes until crispy and golden brown.

6. Add maple syrup and bake for an additional 5 to 10 minutes.

Yield: Serves 4

Per serving: calories 171, fat 4g, sodium 228mg, fiber 6g, protein 7g

Indian Chickpeas

SIDE DISH / SNACK / VEGETARIAN

Bright and colorful, made with turmeric and ginger, both natural anti-inflammatory spices, pair this recipe with curried rice or fresh naan bread to pick up the leftover sauces.

INGREDIENTS

- 1 (16 oz.) can or 1 pound chickpeas

- ½ cup low-sodium vegetable stock

- 2 onions sliced

- 4 T oil

- 1½ tsp turmeric

- ¾ T fresh ginger root or ¼ tsp powdered ginger

- 6 mint leaves

- ½ tsp chili powder

- 2 tomatoes

- salt to taste

- 1 lemon

DIRECTIONS

1. Cook onion in oil, adding turmeric, ginger, mint, chickpeas, then chili, stock, and tomatoes.

2. Cook 10 to 12 minutes, add salt.

3. Add the juice of a lemon or serve with lemon slices.

Calories

Per recipe: 2310 cal., 100g. protein, 79 g. fat (8 sat., 41 poly.)

for 6 servings, 390 calories per serving."

Lima Bean Stew

MAIN DISH / VEGETARIAN

Lima beans will become a favorite in this simple, creamy stew. Many often still stick to the "meat and potatoes" lifestyle. Change your paradigm and start thinking "beans and vegetables." There are so many easy and delicious meals that combine beans and veggies. Globally, beans and vegetables are staples – so eat your way around the world from your very own kitchen.

INGREDIENTS

• 1 (8 oz.) can of lima beans, undrained or 1 cup dried lima beans, cooked

• 2 cups low-sodium vegetable stock

- 2 carrots, sliced

- 2 onions, sliced

- 2 tbsp minced parsley

- 1 tsp peppercorns to taste

- 2 tbsp whole-wheat flour

- 2 cups soy or almond milk

DIRECTIONS

1. Empty beans and vegetable stock into a large pan.

2. Add all other ingredients except the flour and milk and simmer for 1 hour or more until the beans are very soft.

3. Make a paste of the flour and a little cold milk.

4. Heat the rest of the milk to scalding, and stir in flour paste. Cook and stir until thick.

5. Run the bean soup through a strainer or put it through a food processor and combine it with the milk mixture just before serving, adjusting seasoning to taste.

Black Bean Soup

APPETIZER / MAIN DISH / SIDE DISH / VEGETARIAN

This exceptional Black Bean Soup is perfect for chilly fall and winter evenings. It makes a perfect appetizer or main dish. And of course, it is always better the next day.

INGREDIENTS

- 1lb. dried black beans

- 3 quarts water (2 cups to a pint, 2 pints to a quart)

- 2 bay leaves

- ½ – 1 cup of extra virgin olive oil

- 1-2 large red bell peppers seeded and chopped

- 2 shallots, chopped

- 1-2 onions, chopped

- 8 cloves garlic, chopped

- 1 T ground cumin

- 2 T dried oregano

- 1 T sugar

- 2 T salt

- 1 red onion, diced, for garnish (optional)

- 8 oz. sour cream, for garnish (optional)

DIRECTIONS

1. Place the beans in a nonreactive pan. Cover with the 3 quarts of water, add the bay leaves, and bring to a boil. Reduce the heat and simmer the beans for 2 ½ to 3

hours, stirring frequently and adding more water if necessary to keep them well covered.

2. Meanwhile, heat the olive oil in a sauté pan or skillet. Sauté the bell peppers, shallots, and onions over medium heat until the onions are translucent (about 15 minutes)

3. Add the garlic, cumin, dried oregano and sauté for an additional 2 minutes

4. Remove from the heat and let cool slightly

5. When the beans are almost tender, add the onion/pepper mixture, sugar, and salt to the beans and cook until just tender (20 to 30 minutes)

Adjust the seasonings, garnish with the red onion and sour cream, and serve.

Lia Miller's Black Bean Soup, (adapted from Gloria's black bean soup)

Creamy Squash and Bean Soup

MAIN DISH / VEGETARIAN

The Nicoyan diet is based off a foundation of squash, corn, and beans. In a creamy winter twist of corn, squash, and beans, this recipe combines squash and beans, making it rich in complex carbohydrates and protein. All variations of squash that work for this recipe belong to the botanical family Cucurbitaceae, known for providing high levels of useful carotenoids.

INGREDIENTS

• 1 (15 oz.) can navy beans undrained, or 1 pound dried beans, cooked

- 2 cups low-sodium vegetable stock

- 2 lbs Hubbard, butternut, or other hard yellow squash, peeled and cubed

- 2 tbsp olive oil

- 1 pint unsweetened coconut milk (light)

- pepper to taste

- 1 dollop tofu cream (optional)

DIRECTIONS

1. Cook squash in oil in covered pan over low heat.

2. Put both beans and squash through food processor or potato ricer, and return puree to vegetable stock.

3. Add milk, season with pepper and serve very hot.

Heirloom Bean Salad with Smoky Sun-Dried Tomato Vinaigrette

MAIN DISH / SIDE DISH / VEGETARIAN / PLANT-BASED

The longest-lived people in the world eat about a cup of beans every day, and beans are the cornerstone of the Blue Zones diet. This smoky heirloom bean salad recipe is healthy and delicious, perfect for potlucks, parties, and busy weeks.

Yield: 6 servings

INGREDIENTS

7 oz each cooked Black Turtle beans, Hopi lima beans, French navy beans, small red beans, pinto beans, yellow

peas, and green lentils (any combination of dried legumes will work)

2 cups grated Brussels sprouts

1 cup tri-color or red quinoa

5 whole bay leaves

3 tablespoons sea salt

2 tablespoons mushroom base

1 tablespoon thyme

Cilantro, parsley, or fresh scallion, to garnish

SMOKY VINAIGRETTE INGREDIENTS

1 cup grapeseed oil

½ cup sun-dried tomato

⅓ cup white balsamic vinegar

2 tablespoons smoked paprika

2 tablespoons honey

1 tablespoon ground basil

1 tablespoon ground black pepper

DIRECTIONS

1. Soak legumes for 8 hours prior to cooking.

2. Cook quinoa by boiling in 1 quart of water with mushroom base until the quinoa sprouts. Strain excess liquid and spread onto a baking sheet to cool.

3. Cook legumes for 1½-2 hours in one gallon of rapidly boiling water with sea salt, thyme, and bay leaves, skimming foam occasionally. The largest legumes should be al dente. Strain excess liquid and spread onto a baking sheet to cool.

4. Layer ingredients in a large glass or bowl: quinoa, then grated brussels sprouts, then legumes.

SMOKY VINAIGRETTE DIRECTIONS

1. In a food processor or heavy duty blender, process sun-dried tomato with grapeseed oil until smooth.

2. Add white balsamic vinegar to the tomato-oil mixture and process until emulsified.

3. Add honey, sea salt, ground basil, ground black pepper, and smoked paprika and process until evenly distributed.

4. Drizzle 2 tablespoons of the vinaigrette mixture onto the salads; preserve the rest for future use. Garnish with cilantro, parsley, or fresh scallion (optional).

'Ulu Curry Corn Chowder

VEGETARIAN / PLANT-BASED / VEGAN

This tropical twist on corn chowder uses breadfruit ('ulu) a tree fruit similar to jackfruit. 'Ulu has a mild flavor and the consistency of potatoes or taro, but it is higher in protein, fiber, and nutrients. As a staple food in Hawaii, the Caribbean, South Asia, and Polynesia it has become a versatile and easy to use ingredient in many different cuisines. You can find it in Caribbean, Hawaiian, and some Asian grocery stores, or canned at online grocers like Amazon.

Yield: 2-4 servings

INGREDIENTS

2 tablespoons extra virgin olive oil

¼ teaspoon coriander seeds

½ white onion, diced

2 cloves garlic

¼ teaspoon yellow curry powder

1 cup corn

2 cups coconut milk

1 cup precooked 'ulu (Hawaiian breadfruit)*

Sea salt, to taste

¼ cup water

DIRECTIONS

1. Heat oil in a skillet on medium heat and add coriander seeds. Sauté seeds until fragrant.

2. Add onions and garlic and sauté until almost tender.

3. Turn heat up to high and add yellow curry powder, corn, coconut milk, and 'ulu.

4. Bring to a boil and then turn down and let simmer on medium-low until sauce begins to thicken and 'ulu is tender.

5. Add water if sauce thickens too much for your taste. Finish with sea salt and serve.

*Note: If 'ulu is not available, use jackfruit, diced sweet potatoes, or another starchy vegetable.

Dan's Longevity Dal Palak (Spinach Dal)

MAIN DISH / VEGETARIAN / PLANT-BASED / VEGAN

Centenarians in the blue zones eat about a cup of beans every day and often consume a handful of fresh vegetables or greens from their kitchen gardens. Beans and greens are two of the top Blue Zones longevity foods because they feed good bacteria in your gut. Dan Buettner developed this spinach dal recipe to feature both.

Yield: 4 servings

INGREDIENTS

1 cup lentils

1 teaspoon garam masala

1 teaspoon turmeric

1 teaspoon salt

1 can (15 ounces) chopped tomatoes

⅓ cup oil

1 onion, chopped

4 – 5 cloves garlic, separated, chopped finely

1 inch ginger root, chopped

1 teaspoon red pepper flakes

1 cup spinach

2½ cups water

Salt to taste

DIRECTIONS

1. Sauté all spices and vegetables, except spinach, until onions are clear.

2. Add tomatoes, lentils, and water and simmer for 30 mins.

3. Add spinach and cook for 3 more minutes. Salt to taste.

4. Serve over rice or, if you want an extra longevity

Made in the USA
Middletown, DE
12 September 2021